# FAST LIKE A GIRL RECIPES BOOK

A Woman's Guide to Fasting for Fat Burn, Energy Boost, and Hormone Balance

## MICHAEL JUNIOR

**Copyright©2023 Michael J. Patel**

All right reserved

# TABLE OF CONTENT

# INTRODUCTION

Welcome to the book "Fast Like a Girl Recipes Book: A Woman's Guide to Fasting for Fat Burn, Energy Boost, and Hormone Balance."

This transforming recipe book is more than simply a culinary adventure; it's a comprehensive approach to well-being designed exclusively for women.

This guide extends beyond the kitchen, delivering a roadmap to unleashing energy and achieving holistic health. It is packed with a handpicked variety of dishes designed to harness the wonderful advantages of fasting.

You'll find a treasure trove of recipes precisely prepared to inspire women on their wellness journey in these pages.

Each meal, from metabolism-boosting morning rituals to hormone-balancing feasts, is a celebration of flavor and a tribute to fasting's enormous potential as a tool for fat burning, enhanced energy levels, and hormonal balance.

As you explore these recipes, you'll discover not just a roadmap to sustaining your body, but also a route to self-discovery and empowerment. The advantages extend beyond the kitchen, touching on parts of life that are particularly appealing to women.

Accept your path, accept your strength, and discover the keys to a healthier, more vibrant self. Fast like a lady and experience the flavor of total well-being.

# FAST LIKE A GIRL RECIPES BOOK

## Pesto Zoodle Bowl with Grilled Salmon

**Scenario:**
After a day of work or a rejuvenating workout, treat yourself to a wholesome and flavorful meal with this Pesto Zoodle Bowl featuring succulent grilled salmon.

It's a perfect blend of nutrient-packed ingredients that not only satisfies your taste buds but also nourishes your body.

**Ingredients:**
- 1 zucchini, spiralized into zoodles
- 1 salmon fillet
- 2 tablespoons homemade or store-bought pesto sauce
- Cherry tomatoes, halved
- Parmesan cheese (optional, for garnish)
- Salt and pepper to taste
- Olive oil for grilling

**Preparation:**
1. **Grill the Salmon:**
    - Preheat the grill to medium-high heat.

- Brush the salmon fillet with olive oil and season with salt and pepper.
- Grill the salmon for 4-5 minutes per side or until it flakes easily with a fork. Set aside.

2. **Prepare the Zoodles:**
   - Spiralize the zucchini into noodles using a spiralizer.
   - In a pan, sauté the zoodles with a touch of olive oil for 2-3 minutes until they are just tender.

3. **Assemble the Bowl:**
   - Place the sautéed zoodles in a bowl as the base.
   - Top with grilled salmon, cherry tomatoes, and a generous dollop of pesto sauce.
   - Optionally, sprinkle with Parmesan cheese for added flavor.

4. **Garnish and Serve:**
   - Garnish with fresh herbs or a drizzle of extra virgin olive oil for a finishing touch.
   - Serve the Pesto Zoodle Bowl immediately, allowing the warm salmon to complement the fresh zoodles.

**Benefits:**

1. **Rich in Omega-3 Fatty Acids:** Salmon is an excellent source of omega-3 fatty

acids, promoting heart health and reducing inflammation.

2. **Nutrient-Dense Zucchini Noodles:** Zucchini is low in calories and rich in vitamins and minerals, providing a healthy alternative to traditional pasta.
3. **Packed with Antioxidants:** Pesto sauce, made with basil, pine nuts, and olive oil, contains antioxidants that support overall health and well-being.
4. **Low-Carb and High-Protein:** This bowl is low in carbohydrates and high in protein, making it a great option for those looking to maintain a balanced diet.

## Application:

- Enjoy this Pesto Zoodle Bowl with Grilled Salmon as a post-workout meal to replenish your energy levels.
- Make it a part of your weekly meal prep for a quick and nutritious lunch or dinner option.
- Impress your guests by serving this dish at a dinner party; it's not only delicious but also visually appealing.

Indulge in the delightful combination of fresh zoodles, grilled salmon, and flavorful pesto for a meal that caters to your taste, health, and lifestyle.

# Spaghetti Squash with Tomato Basil Sauce

**Scenario:**
Embark on a culinary adventure with this Spaghetti Squash with Tomato Basil Sauce—a healthy, low-carb alternative to traditional pasta dishes.

The natural sweetness of spaghetti squash pairs perfectly with a vibrant tomato basil sauce, creating a satisfying and nutritious meal for any occasion.

**Ingredients:**
*For the Spaghetti Squash:*
- 1 medium-sized spaghetti squash
- Olive oil for drizzling
- Salt and pepper to taste

*For the Tomato Basil Sauce:*
- 2 tablespoons olive oil
- 3 cloves garlic, minced
- 1 can (28 oz) crushed tomatoes
- 1 teaspoon dried oregano
- 1 teaspoon dried basil
- Salt and pepper to taste
- Fresh basil leaves for garnish
- Grated Parmesan cheese (optional)

**Preparation:**
1. **Prepare the Spaghetti Squash:**
    - Preheat the oven to 375°F (190°C).
    - Cut the spaghetti squash in half lengthwise and scoop out the seeds.
    - Drizzle the cut sides with olive oil and season with salt and pepper.
    - Place the squash halves cut-side down on a baking sheet.
    - Roast in the preheated oven for 40-45 minutes or until the flesh is tender and easily pierced with a fork.
2. **Scrape the Squash:**
    - Allow the roasted spaghetti squash to cool slightly.
    - Use a fork to scrape the flesh, creating "spaghetti" strands.
3. **Prepare the Tomato Basil Sauce:**
    - In a saucepan, heat olive oil over medium heat.
    - Add minced garlic and sauté until fragrant.
    - Pour in the crushed tomatoes, dried oregano, dried basil, salt, and pepper.
    - Simmer the sauce for 15-20 minutes, allowing the flavors to meld and the sauce to thicken.

4. **Assemble the Dish:**
   - Spoon the tomato basil sauce over the spaghetti squash strands.
   - Toss the squash and sauce together, ensuring even coating.
5. **Garnish and Serve:**
   - Garnish with fresh basil leaves and, if desired, sprinkle with grated Parmesan cheese.
   - Serve immediately.

**Benefits:**
1. **Low-Carb Alternative:** Spaghetti squash is a nutritious, low-carb substitute for traditional pasta.
2. **Rich in Vitamins:** The squash provides essential vitamins, including vitamin A, C, and B-complex.
3. **Heart-Healthy Olive Oil:** The use of olive oil in both roasting the squash and making the sauce adds heart-healthy monounsaturated fats.
4. **Antioxidant-Rich Basil:** Fresh basil not only adds a burst of flavor but also contributes antioxidants.

**Application:**
- Enjoy Spaghetti Squash with Tomato Basil Sauce as a light and satisfying dinner option.

- Serve it as a side dish alongside grilled chicken or fish for a balanced meal.
- Pack leftovers for a convenient and healthy lunch option.
- Customize the sauce by adding sautéed vegetables or a touch of red pepper flakes for extra spice.

Savor the wholesome goodness of this Spaghetti Squash with Tomato Basil Sauce—a delicious and nourishing alternative that brings a burst of flavor to your table.

# Chia Seed Pudding

**Scenario:**
Embark on a journey of culinary simplicity and nutritional richness with Chia Seed Pudding—an easy-to-make, versatile dish that offers a delightful combination of texture and flavor.

Whether enjoyed for breakfast or as a healthy dessert, this pudding is a testament to the magic of chia seeds and their ability to transform into a delicious and satisfying treat.

**Ingredients:**
- 1/4 cup chia seeds
- 1 cup almond milk (or any milk of your choice)
- 1 tablespoon maple syrup or honey
- 1/2 teaspoon vanilla extract
- Fresh fruits, nuts, or granola for topping (optional)

**Preparation:**
1. **Mix the Base:**
   - In a bowl or jar, combine chia seeds, almond milk, maple syrup (or honey), and vanilla extract.
   - Stir the mixture thoroughly to ensure the chia seeds are well incorporated.
2. **Let It Set:**

- Cover the bowl or jar and refrigerate the mixture for at least 4 hours or overnight.
- During this time, the chia seeds will absorb the liquid and create a pudding-like consistency.

3. **Stir Again:**
   - After the initial setting time, give the chia seed mixture a good stir to break up any clumps and ensure an even texture.

4. **Customize:**
   - At this point, you can add more almond milk if a thinner consistency is desired.
   - Optionally, add sweeteners or flavorings to suit your taste.

5. **Top and Serve:**
   - Serve the Chia Seed Pudding in individual bowls or jars.
   - Top with fresh fruits, nuts, or granola for added texture and flavor.

**Benefits:**

1. **Rich in Omega-3 Fatty Acids:** Chia seeds are an excellent source of omega-3 fatty acids, supporting heart health and overall well-being.
2. **Fiber-Rich:** Chia seeds are packed with soluble fiber, promoting digestive health and providing a feeling of fullness.

3. **Protein-Packed:** Chia seeds contain a good amount of plant-based protein, essential for muscle repair and growth.
4. **Customizable and Nutrient-Dense:** The pudding is highly customizable, allowing you to incorporate a variety of flavors and toppings while providing essential nutrients.

## Application:

- Enjoy Chia Seed Pudding as a wholesome breakfast option, topped with your favorite fruits and a drizzle of honey.
- Serve it as a healthy dessert alternative, garnished with dark chocolate shavings or a dollop of whipped cream.
- Pack it in a portable container for a convenient and nutritious snack at work or on the go.
- Experiment with different flavor variations by adding cocoa powder, cinnamon, or a splash of citrus juice to the base.

Elevate your culinary experience with Chia Seed Pudding—a versatile and nutrient-packed delight that caters to your taste buds and nourishes your body.

# Quinoa Salad with Lemon-Tahini Dressing

**Scenario:**
Embark on a journey of wholesome goodness with this Quinoa Salad with Lemon-Tahini Dressing—a vibrant and nutritious dish that celebrates the versatility of quinoa and the zesty flavors of a delightful homemade dressing.

Perfect as a light lunch or a refreshing side, this salad offers a symphony of textures and tastes that will leave you satisfied and nourished.

**Ingredients:** *For the Quinoa Salad:*
- 1 cup quinoa, rinsed
- 2 cups water or vegetable broth
- 1 cup cherry tomatoes, halved
- 1 cucumber, diced
- 1 bell pepper (any color), diced
- 1/4 cup red onion, finely chopped
- 1/4 cup Kalamata olives, pitted and sliced
- 1/4 cup feta cheese, crumbled (optional)
- Fresh parsley or mint for garnish

*For the Lemon-Tahini Dressing:*
- 1/4 cup tahini
- 2 tablespoons olive oil
- 2 tablespoons fresh lemon juice
- 1 clove garlic, minced

- 1 teaspoon honey or maple syrup
- Salt and pepper to taste
- Water (as needed to thin the dressing)

**Preparation:**
1. **Cook the Quinoa:**
    - In a medium saucepan, combine quinoa and water or vegetable broth.
    - Bring to a boil, then reduce the heat to low, cover, and simmer for 15-20 minutes or until the quinoa is cooked and water is absorbed.
    - Fluff the quinoa with a fork and let it cool.
2. **Prepare the Salad Ingredients:**
    - In a large bowl, combine the cooked quinoa, cherry tomatoes, cucumber, bell pepper, red onion, Kalamata olives, and feta cheese (if using).
3. **Make the Lemon-Tahini Dressing:**
    - In a small bowl, whisk together tahini, olive oil, fresh lemon juice, minced garlic, honey or maple syrup, salt, and pepper.
    - If the dressing is too thick, thin it with water until you reach the desired consistency.
4. **Dress the Salad:**

- Pour the Lemon-Tahini Dressing over the quinoa salad.
- Toss the salad until all ingredients are well coated with the dressing.

5. **Garnish and Serve:**
   - Garnish the Quinoa Salad with fresh parsley or mint.
   - Serve immediately or refrigerate for a couple of hours to allow the flavors to meld.

**Benefits:**

1. **Complete Protein Source:** Quinoa is a plant-based complete protein, providing all essential amino acids.
2. **Nutrient-Rich Vegetables:** The salad is packed with colorful vegetables, offering a range of vitamins, minerals, and antioxidants.
3. **Healthy Fats:** The Lemon-Tahini Dressing contributes healthy fats from tahini and olive oil.
4. **Customizable and Balanced:** This salad is easily customizable, allowing you to add your favorite vegetables or proteins for variety and balance.

**Application:**

- Enjoy Quinoa Salad with Lemon-Tahini Dressing as a light and satisfying lunch option.

- Serve it as a side dish alongside grilled chicken, fish, or tofu for a complete meal.
- Bring it to potlucks or picnics as a nutritious and flavorful contribution.
- Make a large batch for meal prep, enjoying it throughout the week for quick and healthy lunches.

Elevate your taste buds and nourish your body with the goodness of Quinoa Salad with Lemon-Tahini Dressing—a delightful and versatile dish that brings together the best of flavors and nutrition.

# Coconut Chia Seed Smoothie Bowl

## Scenario:

Start your day on a refreshing note or refuel after a workout with this Coconut Chia Seed Smoothie Bowl. It's a delightful blend of tropical flavors and wholesome ingredients that will leave you energized and satisfied.

## Ingredients:

- 1 cup coconut milk
- 3 tablespoons chia seeds
- 1/2 cup pineapple chunks
- Kiwi slices for topping
- Shredded coconut for garnish

## Preparation:

1. **Prepare Chia Pudding:**
   - In a bowl, mix chia seeds with coconut milk.
   - Stir well and let it sit in the refrigerator for at least 2 hours or overnight until it forms a thick pudding-like consistency.
2. **Blend the Smoothie:**
   - In a blender, combine pineapple chunks and half of the prepared chia pudding.

- Blend until smooth, adding more coconut milk if needed.

3. **Assemble the Bowl:**
   - Pour the pineapple-chia smoothie into a bowl.
   - Top with the remaining chia pudding, kiwi slices, and a sprinkle of shredded coconut.

4. **Garnish and Serve:**
   - Garnish with additional kiwi slices and shredded coconut for a burst of freshness and texture.
   - Serve the Coconut Chia Seed Smoothie Bowl immediately to enjoy its vibrant flavors.

**Benefits:**

1. **Hydration and Electrolytes:** Coconut milk is hydrating and contains natural electrolytes, making it a perfect base for a post-workout smoothie bowl.

2. **Fiber-Rich Chia Seeds:** Chia seeds are an excellent source of fiber, promoting digestion and providing a feeling of fullness.

3. **Vitamin C Boost from Pineapple and Kiwi:** Pineapple and kiwi are rich in vitamin C, supporting immune function and providing antioxidants.

4. **Healthy Fats:** Coconut milk and chia seeds contribute healthy fats that can

support brain health and keep you satiated.

## Application:
- Kickstart your morning with this Coconut Chia Seed Smoothie Bowl as a nutritious and visually appealing breakfast option.
- Use it as a post-exercise recovery meal to replenish energy stores and support muscle recovery.
- Customize the toppings with your favorite fruits, nuts, or seeds to add variety and cater to your taste preferences.
- Impress guests with a tropical-themed brunch by serving these smoothie bowls in decorative bowls, allowing everyone to customize their toppings.

Enjoy the goodness of coconut, chia seeds, and tropical fruits in every spoonful of this delightful smoothie bowl. It's a versatile and nourishing dish that can easily become a staple in your healthy eating routine.

# Mushroom and Spinach Omelette

**Scenario:**
Kickstart your day with a savory and nutrient-packed Mushroom and Spinach Omelette. This quick and easy breakfast option is not only delicious but also provides a healthy dose of protein and essential vitamins to fuel your morning.

**Ingredients:**
- 2 large eggs
- 1/2 cup sliced mushrooms
- Handful of fresh spinach leaves
- 1/4 cup shredded cheese (cheddar, feta, or your choice)
- Salt and pepper to taste
- 1 tablespoon olive oil
- Optional: Chopped herbs like parsley or chives for garnish

**Preparation:**
1. **Prepare the Filling:**
   - Heat olive oil in a pan over medium heat.
   - Add sliced mushrooms and sauté until they release their moisture and become golden brown.

- Add fresh spinach and cook until wilted. Season with salt and pepper. Set aside.

2. **Whisk the Eggs:**
   - In a bowl, whisk the eggs until well beaten.
   - Season with salt and pepper to taste.

3. **Cook the Omelette:**
   - Heat a non-stick skillet over medium heat and add a bit of olive oil.
   - Pour the whisked eggs into the pan, ensuring an even spread.
   - As the edges start to set, lift them slightly with a spatula to let the uncooked eggs flow underneath.

4. **Add the Filling:**
   - Once the omelette is mostly set but still a little runny on top, spread the mushroom and spinach filling over one half of the omelette.
   - Sprinkle the shredded cheese on top.

5. **Fold and Serve:**
   - Carefully fold the other half of the omelette over the filling.
   - Allow it to cook for an additional minute until the cheese melts and the omelette is cooked through.

- Slide the omelette onto a plate, garnish with chopped herbs if desired, and serve hot.

**Benefits:**
1. **High-Quality Protein:** Eggs are a fantastic source of high-quality protein, supporting muscle maintenance and helping you feel full.
2. **Nutrient-Rich Vegetables:** Mushrooms and spinach add a variety of vitamins and minerals, including vitamin D, iron, and folate.
3. **Healthy Fats:** Olive oil contributes heart-healthy monounsaturated fats, providing a satiating element to your breakfast.
4. **Versatile and Low-Carb:** This omelette is low in carbohydrates, making it suitable for those following a low-carb or keto diet.

**Application:**
- Enjoy this Mushroom and Spinach Omelette as a quick and nutritious breakfast, ensuring you start your day with a protein-packed meal.
- Serve it with a side of whole-grain toast or avocado for a more substantial breakfast.
- Customize the omelette by adding other vegetables, herbs, or your favorite cheese.

- Make it a part of your weekend brunch repertoire, impressing friends and family with a delicious and healthy dish.

Elevate your breakfast routine with this Mushroom and Spinach Omelette – a delightful combination of flavors and nutrients in a simple and satisfying package.

# Cucumber Avocado Gazpacho

**Scenario:**
Cool off on a warm day with a refreshing Cucumber Avocado Gazpacho. This chilled soup is not only hydrating but also bursting with the flavors of fresh vegetables and creamy avocado, making it a perfect summer treat.

**Ingredients:**
- 2 large cucumbers, peeled and diced
- 1 ripe avocado, peeled and pitted
- 1 cup cherry tomatoes, halved
- 1/2 red onion, finely chopped
- 1 clove garlic, minced
- 1/4 cup fresh cilantro, chopped
- 2 cups vegetable broth, chilled
- 2 tablespoons lime juice
- Salt and pepper to taste
- Optional: Drizzle of olive oil for garnish

**Preparation:**
1. **Prepare the Vegetables:**
   - Peel and dice the cucumbers.
   - Halve the cherry tomatoes.
   - Finely chop the red onion.
   - Peel and pit the avocado.
2. **Blend the Soup:**
   - In a blender, combine the diced cucumbers, avocado, cherry

tomatoes, red onion, minced garlic, and cilantro.
- Add chilled vegetable broth and lime juice.
- Blend until smooth.

3. **Season and Chill:**
   - Season the gazpacho with salt and pepper to taste.
   - Refrigerate the soup for at least 2 hours to allow the flavors to meld and the soup to chill.

4. **Serve and Garnish:**
   - Ladle the chilled gazpacho into bowls.
   - Drizzle with a touch of olive oil for added richness.
   - Garnish with additional cilantro if desired.

**Benefits:**
1. **Hydration:** Cucumbers and tomatoes have high water content, contributing to hydration and helping you stay cool on hot days.
2. **Healthy Fats:** Avocado provides monounsaturated fats, supporting heart health and enhancing the creaminess of the gazpacho.
3. **Rich in Antioxidants:** The combination of colorful vegetables offers a variety of antioxidants that help combat oxidative stress and promote overall well-being.

4. **Low-Calorie and Nutrient-Dense:** Gazpacho is a low-calorie option packed with essential vitamins and minerals, making it a nutritious addition to your diet.

## Application:

- Serve Cucumber Avocado Gazpacho as a refreshing appetizer at summer gatherings or as a light lunch.
- Pair it with a side of crusty whole-grain bread or a quinoa salad for a more substantial meal.
- Customize the garnishes with a sprinkle of chili flakes or a dollop of Greek yogurt for added flavor and texture.
- Impress guests with the vibrant presentation of this chilled soup in elegant bowls or glasses during outdoor brunches or dinners.

Enjoy the crisp and cool flavors of this Cucumber Avocado Gazpacho as a delightful and nutritious addition to your summer menu.

# Cabbage and Chicken Stir-Fry

## Scenario:
Whip up a quick and nutritious meal with this Cabbage and Chicken Stir-Fry. Bursting with vibrant colors and flavors, this dish offers a perfect balance of lean protein and crunchy vegetables, making it an ideal option for a wholesome dinner or lunch.

## Ingredients:
- 1 pound chicken breast, thinly sliced
- 4 cups shredded cabbage
- 1 carrot, julienned
- 1 bell pepper, thinly sliced
- 2 tablespoons soy sauce
- 1 tablespoon oyster sauce
- 1 tablespoon sesame oil
- 1 clove garlic, minced
- 1 teaspoon ginger, grated
- 2 green onions, sliced
- Sesame seeds for garnish
- Cooked brown rice or quinoa for serving

## Preparation:
1. **Marinate the Chicken:**
   - In a bowl, combine sliced chicken with soy sauce and let it marinate for at least 15 minutes.

2. **Stir-Fry the Chicken:**
   - Heat a wok or large skillet over medium-high heat.
   - Add a bit of sesame oil and stir-fry the marinated chicken until cooked through. Remove from the pan and set aside.
3. **Cook the Vegetables:**
   - In the same pan, add a bit more sesame oil if needed.
   - Sauté garlic and ginger until fragrant.
   - Add shredded cabbage, julienned carrot, and sliced bell pepper.
   - Stir-fry the vegetables until they are tender yet still crisp.
4. **Combine and Season:**
   - Add the cooked chicken back to the pan with the vegetables.
   - Pour in oyster sauce and toss everything together until well combined.
   - Adjust seasoning with additional soy sauce if needed.
5. **Serve and Garnish:**
   - Serve the stir-fry over cooked brown rice or quinoa.
   - Garnish with sliced green onions and sesame seeds for added flavor and texture.

**Benefits:**
1. **High-Quality Protein:** Chicken breast provides lean protein, supporting muscle health and keeping you feeling satisfied.
2. **Fiber-Rich Vegetables:** Cabbage, carrots, and bell peppers contribute dietary fiber, promoting digestive health and providing a range of essential nutrients.
3. **Low in Calories and Healthy Fats:** This stir-fry is low in calories and uses heart-healthy sesame oil, offering a well-balanced and nutritious meal.
4. **Versatile and Quick:** This dish is easily customizable with your favorite vegetables and can be prepared in a short amount of time, making it a convenient option for busy days.

**Application:**
- Enjoy Cabbage and Chicken Stir-Fry as a standalone meal for a light and nutritious dinner.
- Pack leftovers for a flavorful and satisfying lunch the next day.
- Include this dish in your weekly meal prep for a quick and healthy option during busy weekdays.
- Impress guests with a colorful and delicious stir-fry at casual gatherings or potluck dinners.

Elevate your stir-fry game with this Cabbage and Chicken Stir-Fry, a delicious and nutritious combination that's sure to become a staple in your recipe repertoire.

# Sweet Potato and Black Bean Chili

**Scenario:**

Savor the warmth and comfort of a hearty bowl of Sweet Potato and Black Bean Chili. This vegetarian dish is not only flavorful and satisfying but also brimming with wholesome ingredients that make it a perfect choice for a nourishing dinner or a cozy meal on a chilly day.

**Ingredients:**

- 2 large sweet potatoes, peeled and diced
- 1 can (15 oz) black beans, drained and rinsed
- 1 can (14 oz) diced tomatoes
- 1 onion, finely chopped
- 2 cloves garlic, minced
- 1 bell pepper, diced
- 1 jalapeño, seeded and finely chopped (optional for heat)
- 2 cups vegetable broth
- 2 tablespoons chili powder
- 1 tablespoon ground cumin
- 1 teaspoon smoked paprika
- Salt and pepper to taste
- Olive oil for cooking
- Fresh cilantro and lime wedges for garnish
- Optional toppings: Avocado slices, shredded cheese, sour cream

**Preparation:**
1. **Sauté Aromatics:**
   - In a large pot, heat olive oil over medium heat.
   - Add chopped onion and sauté until translucent.
   - Stir in minced garlic and jalapeño (if using) and cook for an additional minute.
2. **Add Sweet Potatoes and Spices:**
   - Add diced sweet potatoes to the pot and cook for about 5 minutes until they start to soften.
   - Sprinkle chili powder, ground cumin, smoked paprika, salt, and pepper over the vegetables. Stir to coat.
3. **Combine Beans and Tomatoes:**
   - Pour in the black beans, diced tomatoes, and vegetable broth.
   - Bring the chili to a simmer and let it cook for 20-25 minutes until the sweet potatoes are tender.
4. **Adjust Seasoning and Serve:**
   - Taste the chili and adjust the seasoning if needed.
   - Serve the Sweet Potato and Black Bean Chili hot, garnished with fresh cilantro and a squeeze of lime juice.

**Benefits:**
1. **Rich in Fiber:** Sweet potatoes and black beans provide a hearty dose of fiber, promoting digestive health and keeping you feeling full.
2. **Packed with Vitamins and Minerals:** Sweet potatoes are rich in vitamins A and C, while black beans contribute iron, magnesium, and potassium.
3. **Vegetarian and Protein-Rich:** This chili is a great source of plant-based protein from black beans, making it a satisfying option for vegetarians and vegans.
4. **Low in Fat and Calories:** With minimal added fats, this chili is a nutrient-dense and low-calorie option for those aiming to maintain a balanced diet.

**Application:**
- Enjoy Sweet Potato and Black Bean Chili on its own for a filling and nutritious meal.
- Serve it over brown rice or quinoa for added texture and a complete protein source.
- Make a big batch and store leftovers for a quick and flavorful lunch throughout the week.
- Share this vegetarian chili at potlucks or gatherings as a crowd-pleasing, wholesome dish.

Warm up your kitchen and your taste buds with this Sweet Potato and Black Bean Chili, a delightful and nourishing meal that's perfect for any occasion.

# Lemon Garlic Herb Shrimp Skewers

**Scenario:**
Transport yourself to a coastal paradise with the delightful flavors of Lemon Garlic Herb Shrimp Skewers. This dish combines succulent shrimp with zesty lemon, aromatic garlic, and fragrant herbs, creating a perfect balance of freshness and richness.

Whether it's a barbecue, dinner party, or a simple weeknight meal, these skewers are a crowd-pleaser.

**Ingredients:**
- 1 pound large shrimp, peeled and deveined
- Zest and juice of 1 lemon
- 3 cloves garlic, minced
- 2 tablespoons fresh parsley, chopped
- 1 tablespoon fresh thyme leaves
- 2 tablespoons olive oil
- Salt and pepper to taste
- Wooden or metal skewers, soaked if wooden

**Preparation:**
1. **Marinate the Shrimp:**
   - In a bowl, combine shrimp with lemon zest, lemon juice, minced garlic, chopped parsley, thyme leaves, olive oil, salt, and pepper.
   - Toss the shrimp until evenly coated and let them marinate for at least 15-20 minutes.
2. **Skewer the Shrimp:**
   - Preheat the grill or grill pan over medium-high heat.
   - Thread marinated shrimp onto skewers, ensuring they are evenly distributed.
3. **Grill the Skewers:**
   - Place the shrimp skewers on the preheated grill.
   - Grill for 2-3 minutes on each side or until the shrimp turn opaque and develop a slight char.
4. **Serve and Enjoy:**
   - Remove the skewers from the grill and transfer them to a serving platter.
   - Garnish with additional chopped herbs and serve immediately.

**Benefits:**
1. **Lean Protein Source:** Shrimp is a low-calorie, high-protein seafood option that supports muscle maintenance and repair.

2. **Heart-Healthy Fats:** Olive oil contributes monounsaturated fats, which are beneficial for heart health.
3. **Vitamin C Boost:** Lemon provides a refreshing burst of vitamin C, offering immune system support.
4. **Herb Infusion:** Fresh herbs like parsley and thyme not only enhance the flavor but also provide antioxidants and additional nutrients.

## Application:

- Serve Lemon Garlic Herb Shrimp Skewers as an impressive appetizer for gatherings or parties.
- Pair the skewers with a light salad for a refreshing and complete meal.
- Enjoy them as the main course alongside grilled vegetables or a quinoa salad.
- Include these skewers in your summer barbecue lineup for a taste of coastal cuisine.

Experience the vibrant and zesty flavors of the coast with these Lemon Garlic Herb Shrimp Skewers, perfect for any occasion that calls for a touch of seaside elegance.

# Greek Salad with Grilled Chicken

**Scenario:**
Indulge in the fresh and vibrant flavors of the Mediterranean with this Greek Salad featuring succulent Grilled Chicken.

This dish combines crisp vegetables, briny olives, creamy feta, and perfectly grilled chicken to create a satisfying and wholesome meal. Ideal for lunch or dinner, it's a culinary journey to the sun-soaked landscapes of Greece.

**Ingredients:**
*For the Salad:*
- 1 pound boneless, skinless chicken breasts
- 1 head romaine lettuce, chopped
- 1 cucumber, diced
- 1 cup cherry tomatoes, halved
- 1/2 red onion, thinly sliced
- 1/2 cup Kalamata olives, pitted
- 1/2 cup crumbled feta cheese
- Fresh oregano leaves for garnish

*For the Marinade:*
- 3 tablespoons olive oil
- 2 tablespoons red wine vinegar
- 2 cloves garlic, minced

- 1 teaspoon dried oregano
- Salt and pepper to taste

**Preparation:**
1. **Marinate the Chicken:**
   - In a bowl, whisk together olive oil, red wine vinegar, minced garlic, dried oregano, salt, and pepper.
   - Place the chicken breasts in the marinade, ensuring they are well-coated. Marinate for at least 30 minutes.
2. **Grill the Chicken:**
   - Preheat the grill or grill pan over medium-high heat.
   - Grill the marinated chicken for 6-8 minutes per side or until fully cooked and has a nice char.
   - Allow the chicken to rest for a few minutes before slicing it into strips.
3. **Assemble the Salad:**
   - In a large bowl, combine chopped romaine lettuce, diced cucumber, cherry tomatoes, thinly sliced red onion, Kalamata olives, and crumbled feta.
4. **Add Grilled Chicken:**
   - Arrange the grilled chicken strips over the salad.
5. **Drizzle with Marinade:**

- Drizzle some of the remaining marinade over the salad as a dressing.
6. **Garnish and Serve:**
    - Garnish the Greek Salad with fresh oregano leaves.
    - Toss the salad gently to combine all the flavors.
    - Serve immediately.

## Benefits:
1. **Lean Protein:** Grilled chicken provides a lean source of protein essential for muscle health.
2. **Nutrient-Rich Vegetables:** The assortment of vegetables in the salad offers a variety of vitamins, minerals, and fiber.
3. **Healthy Fats:** Olive oil, olives, and feta cheese contribute heart-healthy monounsaturated fats.
4. **Antioxidant Boost:** The salad is rich in antioxidants, especially from colorful vegetables and olives, supporting overall health.

## Application:
- Serve Greek Salad with Grilled Chicken as a refreshing and satisfying lunch or dinner option.

- Pack leftovers in a container for a delicious and nutritious workday lunch.
- Impress guests by serving this salad at barbecues or summer gatherings.
- Customize the salad with additional ingredients like cherry peppers, artichoke hearts, or roasted red peppers for added variety.

Indulge in the taste of the Mediterranean with this Greek Salad featuring Grilled Chicken, a delightful and healthy culinary experience.

# Berry Blast Protein Smoothie

**Scenario:**
Energize your day with a burst of flavor and nourishment by sipping on a refreshing Berry Blast Protein Smoothie. Packed with vibrant berries and a protein punch, this smoothie is not only delicious but also a perfect choice for a quick breakfast, post-workout refuel, or a satisfying snack.

**Ingredients:**
- 1 cup mixed berries (strawberries, blueberries, raspberries)
- 1 scoop protein powder (vanilla or berry-flavored)
- 1 cup unsweetened almond milk
- 1 tablespoon almond butter
- Ice cubes

**Preparation:**
1. **Combine Ingredients:**
   - In a blender, add mixed berries, protein powder, almond milk, and almond butter.
   - If desired, add a handful of ice cubes for a chilled and thicker consistency.

2. **Blend Until Smooth:**
   - Blend the ingredients on high speed until the mixture is smooth and creamy.
   - If the smoothie is too thick, you can add more almond milk until you reach your desired consistency.
3. **Taste and Adjust:**
   - Taste the smoothie and adjust sweetness or thickness by adding more almond butter or berries if needed.
4. **Serve and Enjoy:**
   - Pour the Berry Blast Protein Smoothie into a glass.
   - Optionally, garnish with a few whole berries for a decorative touch.

**Benefits:**
1. **Protein Powerhouse:** The addition of protein powder and almond butter makes this smoothie a great source of protein, essential for muscle repair and satiety.
2. **Antioxidant-Rich Berries:** Mixed berries provide a plethora of antioxidants, contributing to overall health and well-being.
3. **Healthy Fats:** Almond butter adds healthy monounsaturated fats, providing a creamy texture and sustained energy.
4. **Dairy-Free and Low-Calorie:** Using almond milk makes this smoothie suitable

for those who are lactose intolerant, and it's naturally low in calories.

**Application:**

- Kickstart your morning by having the Berry Blast Protein Smoothie as a quick and nutritious breakfast.
- Refuel your body post-workout with this protein-packed smoothie to support muscle recovery.
- Use it as a meal replacement or snack when you need a quick and convenient option.
- Customize the smoothie by adding spinach or kale for an extra nutrient boost without compromising the flavor.

Indulge in the goodness of berries and protein with this Berry Blast Protein Smoothie—a delightful and healthy way to fuel your day.

# Eggplant and Chickpea Curry:

## Scenario:
Transport your taste buds to the aromatic spices of India with this Eggplant and Chickpea Curry. Bursting with flavors, this vegetarian dish combines the creaminess of eggplant with the protein-packed goodness of chickpeas, creating a satisfying and wholesome curry that's perfect for a comforting dinner.

## Ingredients:
- 1 large eggplant, diced
- 1 can (15 oz) chickpeas, drained and rinsed
- 1 onion, finely chopped
- 2 tomatoes, diced
- 3 cloves garlic, minced
- 1 tablespoon ginger, grated
- 1 can (14 oz) coconut milk
- 2 tablespoons curry powder
- 1 teaspoon ground cumin
- 1 teaspoon ground coriander
- 1/2 teaspoon turmeric
- 1/2 teaspoon red chili flakes (adjust to taste)
- Salt and pepper to taste
- Fresh cilantro for garnish
- Cooked basmati rice or naan for serving

## Preparation:

1. **Sauté Aromatics:**
   - In a large pot or deep skillet, heat some oil over medium heat.
   - Add chopped onion and sauté until it becomes translucent.
   - Stir in minced garlic and grated ginger, cooking for an additional minute until fragrant.
2. **Add Spices:**
   - Add curry powder, ground cumin, ground coriander, turmeric, and red chili flakes to the pot.
   - Stir the spices into the onion mixture, allowing them to toast for about a minute.
3. **Cook Eggplant and Chickpeas:**
   - Add diced eggplant and drained chickpeas to the pot, coating them with the aromatic spice mixture.
   - Cook for 5-7 minutes until the eggplant begins to soften.
4. **Pour Coconut Milk:**
   - Pour in the coconut milk, stirring well to combine all the ingredients.
   - Bring the curry to a gentle simmer and let it cook for 15-20 minutes until the eggplant is tender.
5. **Add Tomatoes and Season:**

- Add diced tomatoes to the curry, allowing them to cook for an additional 5 minutes.
- Season the curry with salt and pepper to taste.

6. **Garnish and Serve:**
   - Garnish the Eggplant and Chickpea Curry with fresh cilantro.
   - Serve the curry over cooked basmati rice or with warm naan.

**Benefits:**

1. **Plant-Based Protein:** Chickpeas provide a significant source of plant-based protein, making this curry a nutritious option for vegetarians.
2. **Fiber-Rich Eggplant:** Eggplant adds a hearty dose of fiber, supporting digestion and providing a feeling of fullness.
3. **Healthy Fats from Coconut Milk:** Coconut milk contributes healthy fats, giving the curry a rich and creamy texture.
4. **Antioxidant-Rich Spices:** The blend of curry spices offers antioxidants and anti-inflammatory properties.

**Application:**

- Enjoy Eggplant and Chickpea Curry as a satisfying and complete vegetarian dinner.

- Meal prep the curry for quick and convenient lunches throughout the week.
- Serve the curry at dinner parties or gatherings for a unique and flavorful vegetarian option.
- Customize the spice level to your preference by adjusting the amount of red chili flakes.

Dive into the aromatic world of spices with this Eggplant and Chickpea Curry—a delightful and nutritious journey for your taste buds.

# Lemon-Ginger Detox Water

## Scenario:
Revitalize your body and refresh your senses with this Lemon-Ginger Detox Water. Packed with the cleansing properties of lemon and the soothing warmth of ginger, this infused water is not only hydrating but also a delightful way to kickstart your day or aid in a gentle detox.

## Ingredients:
- 1 lemon, thinly sliced
- 1-inch piece of fresh ginger, peeled and thinly sliced
- 1-2 tablespoons fresh mint leaves
- 1-2 teaspoons honey (optional, for sweetness)
- 4 cups filtered water
- Ice cubes (optional)

## Preparation:
1. **Prepare the Ingredients:**
   - Wash the lemon thoroughly and cut it into thin slices.
   - Peel and thinly slice the fresh ginger.
   - Gather fresh mint leaves.
2. **Assemble the Detox Water:**
   - In a large pitcher, combine lemon slices, ginger slices, and fresh mint leaves.

- Optionally, add honey for a touch of sweetness.

3. **Infuse with Water:**
   - Pour filtered water over the lemon, ginger, and mint in the pitcher.
   - Stir gently to combine the ingredients.

4. **Refrigerate and Infuse:**
   - Cover the pitcher and refrigerate for at least 2 hours, allowing the flavors to infuse into the water.

5. **Serve Over Ice:**
   - When ready to serve, pour the Lemon-Ginger Detox Water over ice cubes for a refreshing and chilled experience.

**Benefits:**

1. **Hydration:** Lemon-Ginger Detox Water is a hydrating option that promotes increased water intake.

2. **Detoxification:** Lemon and ginger are believed to have detoxifying properties that can aid in digestion and support the body's natural detox processes.

3. **Vitamin C Boost:** Lemons are a rich source of vitamin C, providing an immune system boost and promoting healthy skin.

4. **Anti-Inflammatory:** Ginger has anti-inflammatory properties that may help reduce inflammation in the body.

## Application:

- Start your morning with a glass of Lemon-Ginger Detox Water to kickstart your metabolism and rehydrate after a night's sleep.
- Sip on this infused water throughout the day as a refreshing and healthy alternative to sugary drinks.
- Serve it at gatherings or events as a hydrating and flavorful beverage for guests.
- Customize the recipe by adding other herbs like basil or a few slices of cucumber for additional freshness.

Embrace the simplicity and benefits of this Lemon-Ginger Detox Water—a delicious and nourishing addition to your daily routine.

# Mango Tango Salad

## Scenario:
Dance into a burst of tropical flavors with this vibrant Mango Tango Salad. Featuring juicy mangoes, crisp vegetables, and a zesty dressing, this salad is not only a celebration of colors but also a refreshing and nutritious addition to your menu.

## Ingredients:
*For the Salad:*
- 2 ripe mangoes, peeled, pitted, and diced
- 1 cucumber, diced
- 1 red bell pepper, diced
- 1/2 red onion, finely chopped
- 1 cup cherry tomatoes, halved
- 1 avocado, diced
- Fresh cilantro or mint leaves for garnish

*For the Dressing:*
- 3 tablespoons extra-virgin olive oil
- 2 tablespoons lime juice
- 1 tablespoon honey or maple syrup
- 1 teaspoon Dijon mustard
- Salt and pepper to taste

## Preparation:
1. **Prepare the Ingredients:**
    - Peel, pit, and dice the ripe mangoes.

- Dice the cucumber, red bell pepper, red onion, and avocado.
- Halve the cherry tomatoes.

2. **Assemble the Salad:**
   - In a large salad bowl, combine the diced mangoes, cucumber, red bell pepper, red onion, cherry tomatoes, and diced avocado.

3. **Prepare the Dressing:**
   - In a small bowl, whisk together extra-virgin olive oil, lime juice, honey or maple syrup, Dijon mustard, salt, and pepper.

4. **Dress the Salad:**
   - Drizzle the dressing over the salad ingredients.
   - Gently toss the salad to coat evenly with the dressing.

5. **Garnish and Serve:**
   - Garnish the Mango Tango Salad with fresh cilantro or mint leaves.
   - Serve immediately, allowing the flavors to meld.

**Benefits:**
1. **Rich in Vitamins:** Mangoes are a great source of vitamin C, while other vegetables contribute various vitamins and minerals.
2. **Healthy Fats:** Avocado and olive oil add monounsaturated fats, promoting heart health and enhancing satiety.

3. **Hydration:** Cucumber has high water content, contributing to hydration and a refreshing crunch.
4. **Antioxidant Boost:** The combination of colorful fruits and vegetables provides a range of antioxidants, supporting overall health.

## Application:

- Enjoy Mango Tango Salad as a light and refreshing side dish for grilled chicken or fish.
- Serve it as a standalone lunch option, topped with grilled shrimp or tofu for added protein.
- Bring it to picnics or potlucks as a colorful and flavorful contribution.
- Customize the salad by adding a hint of chili powder for a spicy twist.

Embrace the tropical vibes and nutritious goodness of this Mango Tango Salad—a delicious and vibrant dish that's sure to brighten any meal.

# Zucchini Noodles with Pesto

## Scenario:

Embark on a culinary adventure with Zucchini Noodles with Pesto—a light, flavorful, and low-carb alternative to traditional pasta. This dish is not only a celebration of fresh, vibrant ingredients but also a quick and delicious way to enjoy the essence of summer.

## Ingredients:

*For the Zucchini Noodles:*
- 4 medium-sized zucchini
- Salt for sprinkling

*For the Pesto:*
- 2 cups fresh basil leaves, packed
- 1/2 cup grated Parmesan cheese
- 1/2 cup pine nuts, toasted
- 2 garlic cloves, peeled
- 1/2 cup extra-virgin olive oil
- Salt and pepper to taste
- Squeeze of fresh lemon juice (optional)

## Preparation:

1. **Prepare the Zucchini Noodles:**
   - Using a spiralizer or a vegetable peeler, create noodles from the zucchini.
   - Sprinkle the zucchini noodles with salt and let them sit in a colander

for about 15-20 minutes to release excess moisture.
- Afterward, pat the noodles dry with a paper towel.

2. **Make the Pesto:**
   - In a food processor, combine basil leaves, grated Parmesan cheese, toasted pine nuts, and peeled garlic cloves.
   - Pulse until the ingredients are finely chopped.
   - With the food processor running, slowly drizzle in the olive oil until the pesto reaches your desired consistency.
   - Season with salt and pepper. Add a squeeze of fresh lemon juice for brightness if desired.

3. **Toss the Noodles with Pesto:**
   - In a large bowl, toss the zucchini noodles with the freshly made pesto until well coated.

4. **Serve and Enjoy:**
   - Plate the Zucchini Noodles with Pesto and, if desired, garnish with additional Parmesan cheese, pine nuts, or a sprinkle of fresh basil.

**Benefits:**
1. **Low-Calorie and Nutrient-Rich:** Zucchini noodles are a low-calorie

alternative to traditional pasta and provide vitamins and minerals.

2. **Healthy Fats:** The pesto, made with extra-virgin olive oil and pine nuts, adds heart-healthy monounsaturated fats.
3. **Antioxidant Boost:** Basil is rich in antioxidants, promoting overall health and well-being.
4. **Gluten-Free and Keto-Friendly:** This dish is naturally gluten-free and fits well into a keto or low-carb lifestyle.

## Application:

- Serve Zucchini Noodles with Pesto as a light and refreshing lunch or dinner option.
- Pair it with grilled chicken, shrimp, or your protein of choice for a more substantial meal.
- Enjoy it as a cold salad for picnics, potlucks, or as a refreshing side dish during warm weather.
- Customize the pesto by adding spinach, arugula, or a touch of lemon zest for variation.

Experience the joy of guilt-free indulgence with Zucchini Noodles with Pesto—a delightful and healthy twist on a classic pasta dish.

# Avocado and Salmon Nori Rolls

**Scenario:**
Embark on a culinary journey with these Avocado and Salmon Nori Rolls—a fusion of fresh ingredients and delicate flavors. Perfect as a light meal or appetizer, these rolls showcase the harmony of creamy avocado, savory salmon, and the umami richness of nori seaweed.

**Ingredients:**
*For the Nori Rolls:*
- 4 sheets of nori seaweed
- 2 cups sushi rice, cooked and seasoned with rice vinegar, sugar, and salt
- 1 ripe avocado, thinly sliced
- 8 ounces sushi-grade salmon, thinly sliced
- 1 cucumber, julienned
- Soy sauce and pickled ginger for serving
- Sesame seeds and chopped chives for garnish (optional)

**Preparation:**
1. **Prepare the Ingredients:**
   - Cook sushi rice according to package instructions and season it with rice vinegar, sugar, and salt. Allow it to cool.

- Thinly slice the avocado and sushi-grade salmon.
- Julienned the cucumber.

2. **Assemble the Nori Rolls:**
   - Place a sheet of nori on a bamboo sushi rolling mat.
   - Wet your hands to prevent sticking and spread an even layer of sushi rice over the nori, leaving a small border at the top.

3. **Layer Ingredients:**
   - Arrange avocado slices, salmon slices, and julienned cucumber along the bottom edge of the rice.

4. **Roll and Seal:**
   - Carefully lift the edge of the mat closest to you, and roll it over the ingredients, applying gentle pressure to shape the roll.
   - Moisten the top border of the nori with water to seal the roll.

5. **Slice and Garnish:**
   - Using a sharp knife, slice the roll into bite-sized pieces.
   - Optionally, sprinkle sesame seeds and chopped chives over the rolls for garnish.

6. **Serve and Enjoy:**
   - Arrange the Avocado and Salmon Nori Rolls on a platter.

- Serve with soy sauce and pickled ginger on the side.

**Benefits:**

1. **Omega-3 Fatty Acids:** Salmon is rich in omega-3 fatty acids, promoting heart health and providing essential nutrients.
2. **Healthy Fats:** Avocado adds creamy texture and healthy monounsaturated fats.
3. **Fiber and Hydration:** Cucumber contributes fiber and water content, aiding digestion and hydration.
4. **Low-Calorie and Nutrient-Dense:** Nori rolls are a light and nutrient-dense option, making them suitable for a balanced diet.

**Application:**

- Serve Avocado and Salmon Nori Rolls as an elegant appetizer for dinner parties or gatherings.
- Enjoy them as a light lunch or dinner alongside a side salad.
- Include these rolls in a sushi platter for a diverse and visually appealing assortment.
- Customize the fillings with ingredients like mango, crab, or radish for variety.

Savor the delicate flavors and artful presentation of Avocado and Salmon Nori

Rolls—a delightful and nutritious addition to your culinary repertoire.

# Cauliflower Rice Stir-Fry

## Scenario:

Delight your taste buds with this Cauliflower Rice Stir-Fry—a low-carb, veggie-packed alternative to traditional stir-fry. Bursting with colorful vegetables and savory flavors, this dish is not only delicious but also a wholesome option for a quick and nutritious dinner.

## Ingredients:

*For the Cauliflower Rice:*
- 1 large head of cauliflower, washed and trimmed
- 2 tablespoons vegetable oil
- 1 teaspoon garlic, minced
- Salt and pepper to taste

*For the Stir-Fry:*
- 1 cup broccoli florets
- 1 carrot, julienned
- 1 bell pepper (any color), thinly sliced
- 1 cup snap peas, trimmed
- 1 cup tofu or cooked chicken, diced
- 2 tablespoons soy sauce
- 1 tablespoon sesame oil
- 1 tablespoon rice vinegar
- 1 teaspoon ginger, grated
- 2 green onions, sliced
- Sesame seeds for garnish (optional)

**Preparation:**
1. **Prepare Cauliflower Rice:**
   - Cut the cauliflower into florets.
   - Using a food processor or box grater, rice the cauliflower until it resembles rice grains.
   - In a large skillet, heat vegetable oil over medium heat. Add minced garlic and sauté until fragrant.
   - Add cauliflower rice, season with salt and pepper, and stir-fry for 5-7 minutes until tender.
2. **Cook the Stir-Fry:**
   - In the same skillet, add a bit more oil if needed.
   - Add broccoli florets, julienned carrot, sliced bell pepper, and snap peas. Stir-fry for about 5-7 minutes until the vegetables are crisp-tender.
3. **Add Protein and Sauce:**
   - Push the vegetables to one side of the skillet and add tofu or cooked chicken to the other side.
   - In a small bowl, whisk together soy sauce, sesame oil, rice vinegar, and grated ginger. Pour the sauce over the stir-fry and toss everything together.

4. **Finish and Garnish:**
   - Stir in sliced green onions and toss until well combined.
   - Garnish the Cauliflower Rice Stir-Fry with sesame seeds if desired.
5. **Serve and Enjoy:**
   - Divide the stir-fry onto plates and serve immediately.

**Benefits:**

1. **Low-Carb Alternative:** Cauliflower rice is a nutritious, low-carb substitute for traditional rice.
2. **Vegetable Variety:** The stir-fry is loaded with colorful vegetables, providing a spectrum of vitamins and minerals.
3. **Lean Protein:** Tofu or chicken adds a source of lean protein, essential for muscle health.
4. **Heart-Healthy Fats:** Sesame oil contributes healthy fats, enhancing the flavor and providing satiety.

**Application:**

- Enjoy Cauliflower Rice Stir-Fry as a standalone meal for a light and healthy dinner.
- Pack leftovers for a nutritious and convenient lunch option.
- Customize the stir-fry with your favorite vegetables or protein sources for variety.

- Include this dish in your meal prep routine for a quick and satisfying option during busy weekdays.

Embrace the goodness of vegetables and the versatility of cauliflower rice with this flavorful Cauliflower Rice Stir-Fry—a delightful and wholesome addition to your culinary repertoire.

# Turmeric Chicken Skewers

**Scenario:**
Transport your taste buds to a world of vibrant flavors with these Turmeric Chicken Skewers—a fusion of aromatic spices and succulent chicken. Grilled to perfection, these skewers are not only a feast for the senses but also a wholesome and protein-packed addition to your menu.

**Ingredients:**
*For the Marinade:*
- 1.5 pounds boneless, skinless chicken breasts, cut into cubes
- 2 tablespoons plain yogurt
- 1 tablespoon olive oil
- 1 tablespoon ground turmeric
- 1 teaspoon ground cumin
- 1 teaspoon ground coriander
- 1 teaspoon paprika
- 1 teaspoon garlic powder
- 1 teaspoon ginger, grated
- Salt and pepper to taste

*For the Skewers:*
- Wooden or metal skewers, soaked if wooden
- Lemon wedges for serving
- Fresh cilantro for garnish

**Preparation:**
1. **Prepare the Marinade:**
   - In a bowl, combine yogurt, olive oil, ground turmeric, ground cumin, ground coriander, paprika, garlic powder, grated ginger, salt, and pepper.
   - Mix the marinade until well combined.
2. **Marinate the Chicken:**
   - Add the chicken cubes to the marinade, ensuring each piece is coated.
   - Cover the bowl and refrigerate for at least 30 minutes, allowing the flavors to infuse.
3. **Skewer the Chicken:**
   - Preheat the grill or grill pan over medium-high heat.
   - Thread the marinated chicken cubes onto the skewers.
4. **Grill the Skewers:**
   - Grill the chicken skewers for 4-5 minutes per side or until fully cooked and has a nice char.
   - Baste the skewers with any remaining marinade while grilling for added flavor.
5. **Serve and Garnish:**
   - Arrange the Turmeric Chicken Skewers on a serving platter.

- Garnish with fresh cilantro and serve with lemon wedges on the side.

**Benefits:**
1. **Anti-Inflammatory Properties:** Turmeric, the star ingredient, contains curcumin, known for its anti-inflammatory and antioxidant properties.
2. **Protein-Rich:** Chicken is an excellent source of lean protein, essential for muscle health.
3. **Flavorful Spices:** The combination of cumin, coriander, paprika, and ginger adds layers of flavor and additional health benefits.
4. **Grilled and Low-Fat:** Grilling keeps the dish light, and using yogurt in the marinade adds tenderness without excessive fat.

**Application:**
- Serve Turmeric Chicken Skewers as a main course for dinner, accompanied by a side of rice or quinoa.
- Include these skewers in your barbecue lineup for a unique and flavorful option.
- Slice the grilled chicken off the skewers and use it in wraps or salads for a versatile meal.
- Pair the skewers with a yogurt-based dipping sauce for added creaminess.

Transport your palate to a realm of spices and savor the goodness of Turmeric Chicken Skewers—a delightful and wholesome dish that's sure to impress.

# Green Goddess Smoothie

**Scenario:**
Elevate your mornings with the Green Goddess Smoothie—a nutrient-packed, vibrant blend of green goodness that will leave you feeling refreshed and energized. Packed with leafy greens, fruits, and a touch of natural sweetness, this smoothie is a delicious way to kickstart your day.

**Ingredients:**
- 1 cup spinach leaves, packed
- 1/2 cup kale leaves, stems removed
- 1/2 cucumber, peeled and sliced
- 1/2 avocado, peeled and pitted
- 1 green apple, cored and diced
- 1/2 banana, peeled
- 1 cup coconut water or almond milk
- 1 tablespoon chia seeds
- Ice cubes (optional)

**Preparation:**
1. **Prepare the Ingredients:**
   - Wash and prepare all the fresh ingredients.
   - Peel and pit the avocado.
   - Core and dice the green apple.
   - Peel the banana.

2. **Assemble in Blender:**
   - In a blender, combine spinach leaves, kale leaves, cucumber slices, avocado, green apple, banana, and chia seeds.
3. **Add Liquid:**
   - Pour in coconut water or almond milk to help with blending.
   - If a thicker consistency is desired, add ice cubes.
4. **Blend Until Smooth:**
   - Blend the ingredients on high speed until you achieve a smooth and creamy consistency.
5. **Taste and Adjust:**
   - Taste the Green Goddess Smoothie and adjust sweetness or thickness by adding more banana or liquid if needed.
6. **Pour and Serve:**
   - Pour the smoothie into a glass or bowl.

**Benefits:**
1. **Rich in Greens:** Spinach and kale are packed with vitamins, minerals, and antioxidants.
2. **Healthy Fats:** Avocado adds creaminess and healthy monounsaturated fats.
3. **Hydration:** Coconut water or almond milk contributes to the smoothie's liquid base, providing hydration.

4. **Fiber and Omega-3s:** Chia seeds add fiber and omega-3 fatty acids for an extra nutritional boost.

## Application:
- Enjoy the Green Goddess Smoothie as a nutritious breakfast to kickstart your day.
- Sip on it as a post-workout recovery drink for a refreshing boost.
- Pack it in a travel cup for a healthy on-the-go snack.
- Customize the smoothie by adding a scoop of protein powder or a spoonful of Greek yogurt for added protein.

Elevate your mornings with the vibrant and nutritious Green Goddess Smoothie—a delicious blend of greens and fruits to nourish your body and tantalize your taste buds.

# CONCLUSION

As we come to the end of "Fast Like a Girl Recipes Book: A Woman's Guide to Fasting for Fat Burn, Energy Boost, and Hormone Balance," we hope that this gastronomic adventure has left an indelible impression on your quest to better health.

Fasting is more than simply a diet; it is a way of life that enables women to tap into their inherent strength, promote resilience, and attain maximum health.

These dishes have been thoughtfully developed to celebrate the uniqueness of the female body in a symphony of tastes and a dance of nutrients. Aside from the delectable flavors, each meal is an homage to the extraordinary advantages of fasting, which range from improved fat metabolism to increased energy levels and balanced hormones.

Remember that the quest does not end with the final recipe. It pervades your daily life, prompting you to make conscious decisions, embrace self-care, and celebrate your unique power as a woman.

As you enjoy the benefits of this life-changing event, may you continue to fast like a girl - with power, elegance, and the steadfast confidence that you deserve the finest in health and vitality.

**_Cheers to your well-being, strength, and the tasty path ahead!_**